Talk Cancer to Me

Talk Cancer to Me

MY GUIDE TO KICKING CANCER'S BOOTY!

Jessica Lynne DeCristofaro

ISBN: 0692755195
ISBN 13: 9780692755198

Disclaimer

This book is meant as a compilation of my personal experiences, recommendations, and lessons learned throughout my fight against cancer. The suggestions, products, tips, and home remedies found herein are not meant to be used exclusively in treating medical conditions or symptoms thereof. Science and medical technology have advanced significantly in the modern age, and there is no replacement for the medical treatment provided to you by your doctor. I strongly recommend that you discuss with your doctor the use of any products or the implementation of any of the suggestions contained within this book. That being said, and acknowledging that I am a patient, not a doctor, I have found many of these to be of personal benefit, and I share them with you in the hope that they can provide a supplemental benefit to the care that is being provided by your medical doctor.

Table of Contents

Acknowledgments

Thank you to my mother, who gave up her life to be my caregiver and never missed one of my appointments. I couldn't have done this without you. One day I hope to be half the woman you are.

Thank you to my mentor, Ajmal Ali, who always believed in me, even when I didn't believe in myself. I hope this book makes you proud.

Thank you to Christian Tang for supporting my vision and helping it come to fruition.

Thank you to Lorin Levinson, who never missed a day to check in on me.

Thank you to Will and Tamara Hartnett, for giving me hope, when I needed it the most.

Thank you to Myocortex, for helping me get back on my feet again, after my chemotherapy drugs got the best of me. Literally.

Thank you to all of the cancer survivors and fighters out there who gave me the strength I needed to fight. Thank you to all of my friends and family members who have stuck by me throughout this difficult journey. I know it wasn't easy for you, and you gave me something to fight for.

Thank you to my doctors for ultimately saving my life. Especially you, Dr. Izzidore Lossos. You are a genius. Thank you to my favorite nurses, Liezl Root and Vanessa Perez, for everything that you have done for me. Thank you to Dr. Jorge Monge Urrea for helping me overcome the most difficult part of the entire process. There is no doubt in my mind that you are going to make an amazing hematologist one day.

CHAPTER 1

Introduction

Cancer \ kan-ser \ n: 1: A malignant and invasive growth or tumor, especially one originating in epithelium, tending to recur after excision and to metastasize to other sites. 2: Any disease characterized by such growths.*

can-cer \ can-ser \ n: 1: Any disease characterized by a crazy journey/ blessing in disguise that will make you a stronger person and help you realize that you CAN-survive anything life throws at you. This journey will ultimately have you screaming, "Holy crap, what a ride!"

So, you were just diagnosed with cancer. Your initial thoughts are probably somewhere along the lines of "What the hell? Is this a joke?" Or they could be along the lines of "OK, I can handle this." Then one week later, "Seriously, what the hell is going on? Is this really my life?" Those were my initial reactions. But I am here to tell you that yes, it's OK. I am OK, and if I can conquer this, then so can you! That's all you need to realize right now, before you continue reading. Cancer sucks, no matter what type you have, but you *will* get through it, and in the end, it will make you a stronger, much happier person. It won't be easy; it will be a long and difficult journey, but you will get through it, and it will be very rewarding in the end.

---

* Dictionary.com. *Dictionary.com Unabridged*. Random House, Inc. http://www.dictionary.com/brcwse/cancerous. Accessed: July 18, 2016.

Me, Myself, and I

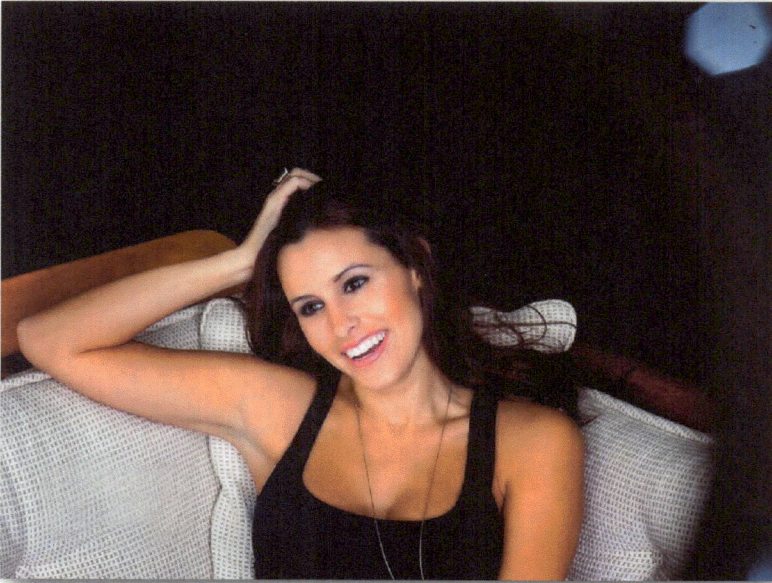

So, let me tell you about myself. My name is Jess. I am twenty-nine years old. I'm originally from Boston, but I relocated to Miami in 2009. I'm a Miami transplant but a New England girl at heart. I'm a sales representative for a major pharmaceutical company. I'm a normal twenty-nine-year-old. I love to socialize with my friends, go out on the town, hang out at the beach, have a few drinks, exercise, hang out with my dog…I could go on and on. I was diagnosed with stage IV nodular sclerosis Hodgkin's lymphoma in February of 2016, at age twenty-eight, shortly before my twenty-ninth birthday. Happy birthday to me, right? It was actually a blessing in disguise.

When you are diagnosed with cancer, your oncologist or hematologist does not give you a guidebook to help you try to understand the weird things that will happen to your mind and body. They treat you with medication, chemotherapy, radiation, and possibly surgery, if indicated, and then throw you back out into the real world. They may give you a small medical pamphlet with bulleted points briefly describing chemo and how to handle it, health guidelines to follow, dietary restrictions, and so forth. Unfortunately, the pamphlet is so concise that you will have many unanswered questions. This is certainly frustrating!

Unfortunately, at the end of the day, you may find that the doctors are so busy that your questions, which are so important to you, are not important to them and remain unanswered. Questions like, "Can I go to my friend's birthday party? Can I drink alcohol? What do I do when people stare at me because they know I have cancer?" These questions, while so important to you, are not equally important to them since their main focus is on curing you as quickly as possible. So, as cancer patients, unless our problems involve new symptoms or a fever, our problems are "first world problems" to them. In hindsight, that makes perfect sense; however, it didn't at the time I was diagnosed, for sure.

After my diagnosis was confirmed, my initial instinct was to go home and do a search on Amazon for books on how to deal with cancer. There are many good books out there—don't get me wrong—they just weren't for me. They weren't appropriate or helpful to my life circumstances. I needed something that would appeal more to someone in my age group, that would help me understand what was happening to me medically and instruct me on how I could deal with the physical and emotional changes and insults to my poor body and mind. I couldn't really find any blogs either, so I decided to create my own. Then I gave some thought to composing a guidebook on how to get through this bad boy and about what truly worked for me. Everyone is different, and things don't work the same for everyone, but this is what worked for me.

Having cancer is extremely difficult. It's one of the hardest things I've faced my entire life, and my goal is to be able to help you get through this too, with as few obstacles in your path as possible!

So let me tell you my story and how I was diagnosed. January 28, 2016, was the day my world was flipped upside down—the day shit truly hit the fan. I was twenty-eight years old, living what I would call a pretty great life. I was at the height of my career and one of the top sales reps in my division at the international pharmaceutical company where I worked. I was traveling every month, having a great time with friends, meeting new people, going out on the town, and truly enjoying myself. I finally felt like I was established and had it all. Little did I know that I was in for a huge wake-up call.

Background Symptoms

Here is the background information that might help you better understand what was happening to my body before lymphoma took over like wildfire. I had been struggling with an annoying, chronic, and lingering cough for two to three years—essentially, around-the-clock coughing. The cough was like a curse; it wouldn't go away. I was examined by multiple doctors, including PCPs, allergists, ENTs, and GI doctors; you name it, and I had been to one. Originally, I had been diagnosed with allergies, so I took allergy medication for approximately one and a half to two years. The cough still wouldn't subside. I remember my friends, my boyfriend at the time, and coworkers advising me to make appointments with several different doctors because something wasn't right. I dismissed these suggestions, because if you see ten doctors, and each tells you the same thing, it's not a big deal. They are probably right, right? Wrong! After having taken allergy medications for almost an entire year, my allergist told me I might have something called acid reflux. She recommended making an appointment with an ENT for an evaluation.

I met with two ENTs, who both told me I had acid reflux. They recommended a specific dietary plan, which I followed; performed an exam to confirm that it was reflux; and prescribed omeprazole (commonly known as the OTC drug Prilosec). The cough subsided for a short time, but then it came back and was worse than it had been previously. They concluded I should probably see a GI doctor who might want to schedule an endoscopy. As November 2015 approached, my cough got incredibly worse. I remember being in Boston visiting my best friends, and I—seriously—could *not* stop coughing. I blamed it on going out the night before and being hungover. Maybe the excessive amount of alcohol was causing the cough, because if you have reflux, you're not supposed to be drinking alcohol. So consuming a few fireball shots a night probably wasn't the best idea—oops. The cough was very bad. When I returned to Miami, I met with two different GI doctors. They *both* told me it was probably reflux, prescribed omeprazole again at a higher strength for a few months, and set up an endoscopy. I was coughing nonstop day and night. So I was set up for an endoscopy mid-February, after I would be returning from my national sales meeting in Vegas as planned.

Here is where my story gets a bit more interesting. Besides the annoying cough, I had other symptoms as well: excruciating abdominal pain, back pain, night sweats, and itchy skin on both of my legs (treated as atopic dermatitis). I religiously started working out with a personal trainer and good friend of mine who owned a studio. Rob and his business partner, Courtney, enrolled me in a customized Pilates and strength-training program. I was in the best shape of my life from working with these two professionals for several months. However, several months into training, I started having severe bouts of abdominal pain. My PCP told me it was from tearing a muscle while working out. He gave me a muscle relaxant and sent me on my way. In the event that the pain was related to my reproductive system, I figured I should probably see my ob-gyn—just a wild guess—because sometimes the pain felt like menstrual cramping. My ob-gyn performed an ultrasound, but everything was negative, and I did not have any ovarian cysts. The diagnosis again was I had probably torn a muscle. I struggled with this pain for months on and off, basically relying on Advil to get me through the days. I can't even tell you how much Advil I popped daily. I also woke up at night drenched in perspiration. I thought it was just because of my increased metabolism from working out so hard.

Little did I know that everything was about to blow up. In January, I developed a giant lump underneath my left armpit. I immediately went to my PCP, who told me it was a cyst. I texted Courtney and told her I couldn't work out because my armpit hurt so badly. It was excruciatingly painful. Then, shortly after that, another lump developed under my right armpit. I didn't think anything of it because I had heard that if you get a cyst under one arm, you usually get one under the opposite arm as well—no worries!

When Things Really Hit the Fan

I had no time to deal with all the crazy symptoms at that point; after all, it was January 28, and I was getting ready to go to the national sales meeting in Vegas on January 30. I was all packed and ready to head out there early to see my friend who lives in LA. She was meeting me in Vegas. Because we were all meeting Saturday in Vegas for a little preparty before the meeting, I was in so many group texts with my girlfriends from work. I could not have been more excited. Unfortunately, the pain that day was unbearable in my abdomen, and believe me, I have extremely high tolerance to pain. I can handle almost anything. I kept making excuses for the cause of the pain—I had been socializing a lot with friends and not getting enough sleep, or maybe I needed to relax a bit and stop partying so much. I stopped at a CVS during work and managed to keep going by using Icy Hot chill-stick compresses while trying to lug my product-sample bag into doctors' offices to drop off samples. I could barely work until noon that day. I figured I should try to get muscle relaxants for what I thought was another horrible muscle tear.

I finally decided to go to an urgent-care center. I sat there for a few hours, and the doctor told me it was probably a muscle tear. Then they told me I had kidney stones. They advised me to go to the hospital, as it was obvious they really did not know how to treat me. I was seriously considering putting off going to the hospital until after I returned from Vegas. Thank God I didn't. I immediately called my mom and told her about my situation. She is an RN and has her PhD in education, so she's a smart cookie, and she advised me to go to the ER. I went to the ER thinking, "OK, maybe kidney stones; give me some pain relievers and send me home." I was wrong for sure! After many hours of waiting, lots of blood work, a CT scan, and a chest x-ray, it was one o'clock in the morning. The doctor came in and told me I needed to be admitted, get more scans, and be seen by more specialists in the morning. The look on his face was blank. My white blood cell count was dangerously high, and more diagnostic tests needed to be performed.

I called my mom, who never freaks out. That's when I knew something was wrong. She knew I was in trouble and insisted I cancel my Vegas trip, have the CT scan done, and have the attending physician call her. She was in NY taking care of her elderly mother, who had fractured her hip. I called one of my girlfriends immediately. She came to the hospital, picked up my keys, and ran to my apartment to get my dog. All I could think about was getting out of there before I had to jump on a flight in one more day. I kept telling all the nurses I had a flight to catch. They just smiled and didn't really say anything because they already knew I wasn't going anywhere.

The Worst Day Ever

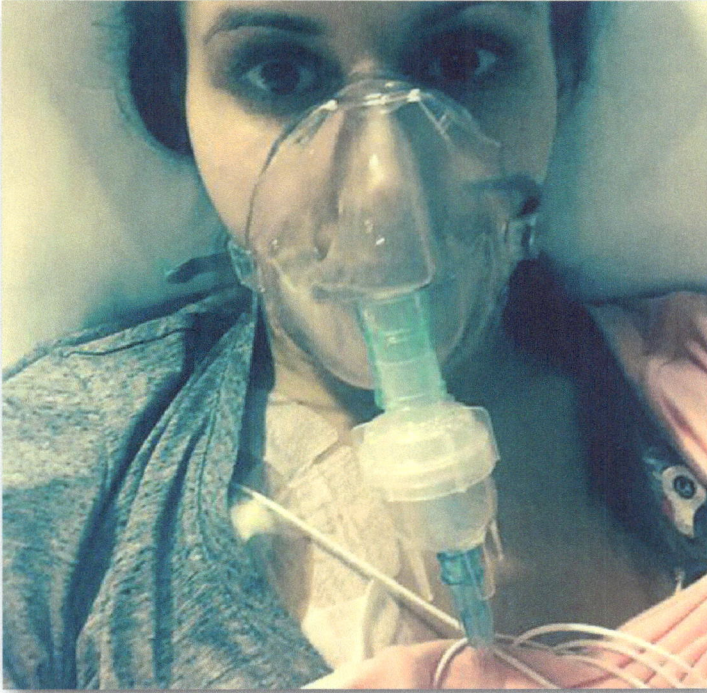

January 29, 2016. Tests. All day. All night. My mom was on a flight en route to Florida from visiting my sick grandmother in New York. As the day wore on, I became even more ill, and the pain became more severe. I had difficulty breathing. CT scans, x-rays, ultrasounds, oxygen, intravenous fluids, antibiotics, nebulizer breathing treatments, and more blood work. My breathing got worse. I called my friends, my coworkers, and even my manager and told him to cancel my Vegas trip. I wasn't going to make it. I knew something was seriously wrong, but at the same time, I was in denial. I thought about how my aunt had passed away the previous year of AML (acute myeloid leukemia). It was déjà vu, like being in the hospital with her before she passed. Having no recollection of time, I recall waking up to see my girlfriend Olivia in my hospital room. She lives in LA and caught a red-eye. I was so in and out of it and so happy to see her, but that's when I knew something was very wrong. I was pretty much sedated the entire time in the hospital, living on Dilaudid (an opioid) for the pain. My friends kept visiting and kept a watchful eye on me. My mom had arrived and met with the two oncologists as well as the general surgeon.

I finally met with two oncologists who both suspected an infection somewhere in my body but said there was a slight chance it could be lymphoma—but not to worry. They'd run more tests; it was probably an infection. I was scheduled for an excision of the lymph node under my left armpit—the larger one, which was causing more pain. The surgery would be early the next morning, after which the surgeon would send the specimen for biopsy to help establish the diagnosis. The female doctor assured me it was most likely an infection. She also told me if it was lymphoma, I should consider freezing my eggs because I might not be able to have children. I'm sorry, what?

I would also need to have a bone-marrow biopsy and a PET scan to help confirm the diagnosis in addition to the lymph-node biopsy, which would take about two to three days to get results on. If the biopsy of the lymph node and the bone marrow were positive for lymphoma, then I would probably require a portacath inserted into my chest so it would be easily accessible for chemotherapy. Yikes! Way too much information to digest!

Surgery went fine—other than my mom seeing the specimen, being aware of the diagnosis before me, and not telling me. Thanks, Mom! Two days later, I had a bone-marrow biopsy, and then several hours after the bone-marrow biopsy, I had a portacath placed in my chest. Several days after all the surgeries, I contracted pneumonia. I was shaking. I had chills and a 103-degree fever. I was sweating profusely and in a lot of pain. The day the oncologists told me my diagnosis was probably the worst day of my entire life. I was sitting in my hospital bed crying, sweating and shaking. I was feverish and attached to oxygen. I couldn't even shower myself, so Olivia had to wash my body and my hair. I couldn't even walk. What the hell? Just the weekend before, I was out with all of my girlfriends having the time of my life; now I was in the ICU? As night approached, all I remember was shaking out of control and Olivia blow-drying my body with her hair dryer to get me to stop shaking. Sorry, Liv. I recently discovered that was not the right protocol, but you tried! Ha!

That night I had to have the nurses change my clothes six times while my friend sat in the hospital chair in my room. I was soaking wet. They told me I had a fever and that it was breaking. Night sweats! I kept telling the nurses I couldn't breathe even with the oxygen, but no one seemed to be listening. They thought it was anxiety and gave me more Ativan, which is absolutely bizarre, considering that would suppress my breathing even more. I really thought at that moment I was going to die, and that was it. I was preparing myself for it. That was a feeling I will never forget. I just kept telling myself in my head, "Don't stop breathing. Don't stop breathing." Finally, after hours of telling the nurses I couldn't breathe, I went into respiratory failure.

Blacking in and out of consciousness, I realized I was in the operating room with my mom next to me. The interventional radiologist withdrew one quart of fluid from my left lung. I looked over and saw two of my neighbors, who are RNs. They had come to see me as well. A few hours later, I could finally breathe.

A bone-marrow biopsy is supposed to be extremely painful, but I was already so messed up on painkillers that I didn't even feel a thing. "Treatment" at the hospital consisted of being blacked out on anxiety and pain medications, and this continued for a week. My friends visited me nonstop, and Olivia caught another red-eye to come see me the following weekend. That's when the news broke: lymphoma. Twenty-eight years old, and I had cancer. I remember two of my friends being in the room when the doctor told me. I was so numb that I couldn't even cry. All I could think about was my pregnant friend, about to pop any day, being told that one of her best friends had cancer, and it absolutely broke my heart. I thought about my mom, who had just lost her sister a year prior to this horrible monster, having to go through this again. I thought about Olivia beside me, who had already lost her sister and her mom, having to go through this too. I thought about all of my other friends and family.

This wasn't just affecting me. It was affecting everyone around me, which scared the crap out of me. But I still didn't cry, because sometimes you have to be strong not only for yourself, but also for the people you love. More friends kept visiting, and it was all becoming very real. All of my close friends came to visit every day. My family friend Ajmal drove several hours to see me, as well as my friend and former client, John, who happens to be a very well known doctor. That's when I knew things must not have been looking too good for me.

My Check-In at the Cancer Center

I was finally diagnosed with stage IV nodular sclerosis Hodgkin's lymphoma. Since it was so aggressive and had spread to multiple organ systems, the oncologists at the hospital weren't prepared to treat me. After waiting a few days for a bed, I was transferred to the ICU at a cancer center. A doctor who deals with high-risk lymphoma cases was going to handle mine. Blacking in and out of consciousness, I just remember waking up to the doctor, his cute resident, and interns, and barely being able to speak. My doctor was absolutely furious that I was in such horrible shape. I work in the health-care industry, and still I'd gone years being misdiagnosed. He scared me. He was upset and frustrated that it had taken almost one week of messing around at the previous hospital without my actually being treated. Chemo would start immediately, as in that evening! I was beyond out of it. I remember one of my doctor's adorable residents calming me down and being so nice.

The doctor chose a regimen of BEACOPP (a chemotherapy regimen for the treatment of Hodgkin's lymphoma with unfavorable risk factors). It's not the standard ABVD lymphoma regimen, but since my cancer was so aggressive, this was the only option for me. BEACOPP is not typically done in the United States, and the doctor even escalated my dosage. Everything was changing in the blink of an eye. Minutes later, medical staff warned me about all the horrible side effects of the chemo I was being treated with: heart disease, lung disease, secondary cancers, infertility, and neuropathy. Since I was stage IV, I also ran a chance of relapse. Unfortunately, I had to be treated right away and did not have time even to think about possible fertility treatments beforehand, and I certainly didn't have time to freeze my eggs. At that point, it was life or death, and obviously, I had to choose life.

Party in the ICU

On the bright side, while in the ICU starting chemo, I met an absolute angel RN named Leizel (also known as Liz). As horrible as this all sounds, she helped me turn a nightmare upside down. Having been at the other hospital for almost two weeks, I'd had many different nurses caring for me on various shifts. The majority of them really didn't care or seem to like their jobs; very few were OK. Liz was the absolute bomb. She had such great energy and always had me laughing. I felt as if I were hanging out in the ICU with one of my girlfriends whom I had known forever. Olivia flew in again and stayed with me that weekend. I just couldn't get over how well she held it together. She was by my side 24-7 and slept in a nasty hospital chair the entire weekend again. She didn't even pack a bag either weekend that she'd flown down; she just jumped on any flight she could get on. If that isn't true friendship, then I don't know what is.

It was Super Bowl Sunday, and I think that's when I realized I had the best friends in the entire world. All of my friends came to see me in the ICU, and we actually had a Super Bowl party while I was on my painkillers. Ha! Leave it to my friends and me to turn a messed-up situation into a party. Scott, a friend who was in town from New York, even spent his Super Bowl night in the ICU. We were all laughing the entire time.

At one point, my friend Lorena came in to break the bad news that it was time to remove my hair extensions! *The end of the world!* Lorena and my former roommate, Kristin, knew it was time. One was on one side of my hospital bed, and one on the other, both ripping out my hair extensions with a fork. Mind you, this was all happening when one of the cute doctors, whom I had apparently been trying to hit on while sedated, was in my room talking to me. Girls, if you are reading this right now, you could have waited until he left the room!

The Chemo Floor

The next day I was doing better and finally transferred out of the ICU and onto the chemo floor. Although it was a horrible situation, and my life was changing right in front of my eyes, I was, in one way or another, happy. I had never felt so loved in my entire life, and I never realized how lucky I was to have such amazing people around me—something many people, including myself, often take for granted. I don't think I could have gotten through those weeks without all my friends. Even people whom I never expected to reach out were coming to visit me in the hospital. I gained new friends and became closer to the ones I already had. My coworkers were absolute angels too. They all pitched in and got me the most amazing cancer kit I could have ever expected to receive. This was filled with books, gift cards, and necessities for my hospital stay. Their support really helped me pull through.

Chemo ended Friday of that week, and it was my last night in the hospital. I was getting discharged Saturday. I was beyond excited. I felt like I was handling the situation pretty well. Since I was being discharged, I also thought it was a great time to stalk down on LinkedIn one of the cute doctors I'd met. I'll call him "Dr. X." I'm a pretty ridiculous person, so this is fitting for the situation. I wrote him a creepy LinkedIn message and tried to get him to come say good-bye before I was discharged. He took me up on my offer and stopped by after one of his night shifts. I had cancer and still had game! Ha, ha! I followed up with another message to him with my phone number. My thinking at that point was, "Screw it! I have cancer and therefore nothing left to lose."

Later that Saturday, I left the hospital with my mask on and was ready to take on the world. I went home quickly to drop off my stuff and went with my mom and cousin to try on wigs, since the doctors said my hair was going to fall out very soon. This was an extremely hard experience since I still had all my hair at that point. I cried a little. But I knew I had to suck it up. Dr. X ended up texting me that night. I still had game, even with cancer!

Home Sweet Home

Next to the night in the hospital thinking I was going to die, the days after I got out were the hardest days of my life. My positive "I can do this" attitude quickly did a 180. I was on so much prednisone that I didn't sleep for almost eight days, was constantly shaking, and felt like an absolute crazy person. Thank God Dr. X was working night shifts and would keep me entertained when I couldn't sleep. I was on my couch day and night just sitting there, looking outside, and crying. I didn't understand what I ever did to deserve this.

My hair started shedding all over my apartment, and that's when my situation became real. I had planned on still working and not taking a leave of absence, because I thought I could handle it. I went into the bathroom and put my hands through my hair, and it fell out in clumps. That's when I really lost my shit. When you have cancer, there are certain moments that you remember—that you will never, ever forget. That's something I will never forget. I took out my hairbrush out, and clump by clump, more hair fell out. I thought I was going to lose my mind. I became sick to my stomach and hung over my toilet dry heaving and crying.

My mom kept telling me this was a good thing because the chemo was working. Every time my hair fell out, she would tell me, don't worry, the chemo is working. I was so sick of her saying this. Being a woman and losing all your hair is probably one of the most traumatizing things anyone can go through. As vain as it sounds, if you have cancer and have lost your hair, you know exactly what I'm talking about. I can't even begin to describe it. Every time some hair would fall out, it made me physically sick to my stomach. And every time it fell out, it was a reminder that what was happening to me was real.

I started having crazy panic attacks after that. One night my mom left to walk my dog for ten minutes. Within those ten minutes, I thought I was going to have a heart attack and stop breathing. I didn't know what to do, so I ran to my neighbors' apartment, pretty much passed out on their floor, and told them to call 9-1-1. I couldn't breathe or talk and just remember putting my mom's cell phone number into my neighbor's phone, telling her to call my mother before I died! They cancelled the 9-1-1 call after they realized I was just having a panic attack. My mom came in two minutes later.

Day by day, my hair kept falling out until there was almost nothing left. I was an emotional wreck. I knew it was time. I called my manager and told him I was going to take a leave of absence from work. After catching up on computer work for a few days, I couldn't bring myself to go in. This was also one of the harder things for me to do—much harder than you could ever imagine. If you knew me, you'd know that I'm all about my career. I'm a very independent, strong woman, and at that moment, I was physically and emotionally weak. I struggled with the decision, but I called my manager in tears, telling him I'd be gone for a bit. He was very supportive about my decision. I knew I had to focus on my health and on getting myself back together.

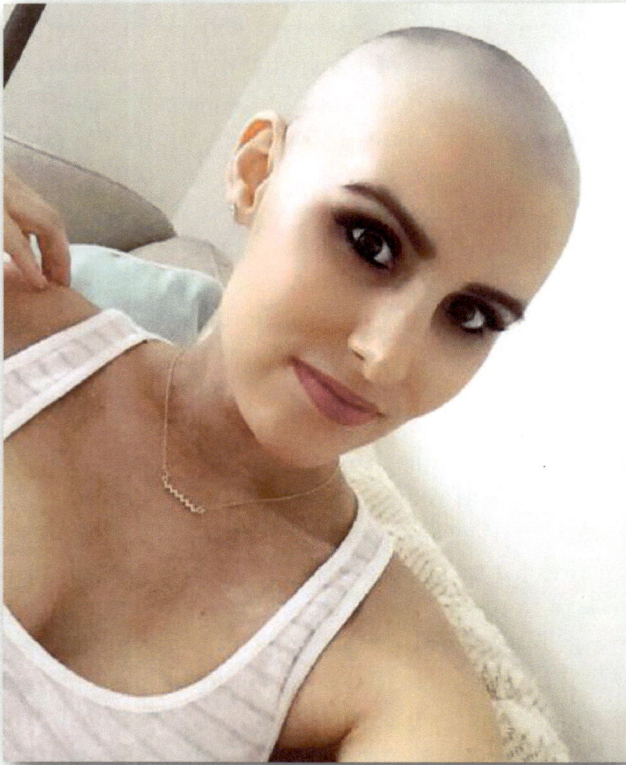

So while this might seem like an extremely depressing introductory story, trust me; it'll get good and entertaining from here. I did eventually get back to my funny, normal self. I'm usually a super private person. My goal here isn't to put my personal life on blast; it is to raise awareness about cancer and to help other people realize that there *is* light at the end of the tunnel and that you're not going through this alone. I remember coming home and googling lymphoma blogs so I could at least have an idea of what to expect, but I couldn't find that many. That was a primary reason for writing this book.

After a few weeks of being miserable, I'd forgotten who I was in the process. I knew it was bad when I didn't even want to call anyone back or answer any messages from friends. I've always been a strong girl, and I've always taken anything that life throws at me with a smile. Always. Life is messy, and crap happens, but at the end of the day, we are forced to deal with it. There is no other choice. These are the cards that I had been dealt, and I had no choice but to deal with them. I am a strong believer that everything in life happens for a reason. I truly believe there is a reason for all this. Maybe I needed to change something in my life, and maybe this small roadblock was going to shake me, wake me up, and help me do that. All I know is that I'm not the same person I was before cancer.

The best advice I've received throughout all of this is that dealing with cancer is 50 percent mental. I truly believe that a lot of it is definitely mental. I turned my time at the ICU into Comedy Central, and I was determined to have the best time possible while I went through chemo, radiation, and so forth, in order to conquer this beast. (Is that possible? Yes! Ask any of my friends. More ridiculous stories to come.) So I picked out a bomb-looking weave (you seriously can't even tell that I have cancer; it's a bit twisted) and put my makeup on every day. I went to my cancer center as if I ran the show, made friends with everyone, hit on the doctors, hung out with my friends when I could, and tried to make life as normal as possible for a few months. It worked for me. Sorry, lymphoma, you messed with the wrong chick!

CHAPTER 2

Talk Chemo to Me

My Chemotherapy Regimen

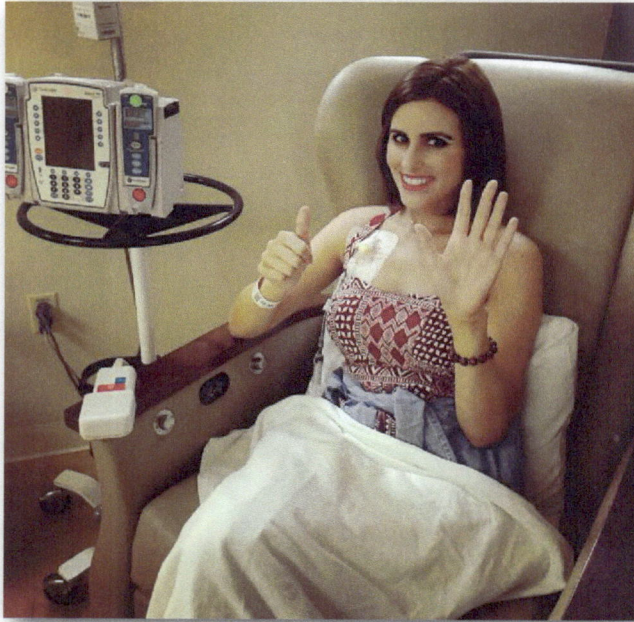

y chemo regimen—escalated BEACOPP—consisted of three straight days of chemo during week one, one day during week two, nothing for week three, and then repeat. I needed a total of six cycles. I'm going to be real with you and tell you how chemo really was for me. I can't tell say whether you will experience the same symptoms, because everyone responds to chemo differently, and all regimens are different.

The first day of the cycle, I got my labs done, visited my doctor, and then went straight to CTU (chemotherapy unit). Basically, I sat there all day in a chair and was blasted with five different chemo drugs through the port in my chest: vincristine, doxorubicin, a cyclophosphamide infusion, etoposide, and prednisone. I'm not really sure what any of these drugs are, Doctor, but my life is in your hands, and I have a lot of things that I still want to do, so please don't mess this up for me! (Seriously, I know I was rude to you in the ICU when we first met. Sorry! I'm going to play the cancer card with that one.) Overall, it's not bad while you're in there, but what *is* creepy is that one of the chemo drugs—I forget which one—is a really strange red color, and it feels weird having all these medications being injected into your body. It's also creepy how you can see everyone else around you getting chemo. People of all genders, ages, and races—all fighting the same battle. I have always been the youngest one so far in my CTU.

I've read so many blogs about experiencing nausea during chemo infusions, which I completely agree with. At the beginning, it wasn't so much the chemo that made me nauseous; it was looking at the other people receiving it. But in a way, seeing this helped me through the process. Many people receiving chemo have terminal cancer. You look around in CTU and see people's aunts, uncles, mothers, fathers, grandparents, and so forth getting their chemo. These are people fighting for their lives, and they don't even stand a chance. I count my lucky stars every night that my cancer wasn't terminal, and even though it always seemed horrible in the moment, it could have been so much worse. I have it good compared to *many* other people. Everyone always tells me that if you're going to have cancer, lymphoma is definitely the one to have. As annoying as this was to hear—since no one enjoys getting chemo or losing their hair—my cancer truly could have been much worse.

The absolute hell began when I got home from chemo. It is imperative to drink as much water as you can and to eat after chemo. Too bad I couldn't eat or drink at first. My mom was practically force-feeding crackers down my throat. The chemo also makes your heart race, so on top of the nausea, I felt like I was going to have a heart attack. I like to call prednisone "predniZONE" because the dose that I received during chemo turned me into a maniac, in the sense that my heart truly felt like it was going to come out of my body 24-7. I am already crazy, so I don't need a medication to contribute to that!

So I spent from about one in the afternoon until five in the morning on my couch dry heaving with a bucket next to me, and my dog sitting there next to me crying. When you get chemo, it kills the good cells and the bad cells in your body, so you basically feel like a zombie. I lost feeling in my fingers, eventually in almost my entire hands, and part of my toes from neuropathy, a side effect of chemo. But hey, at least I still have my fingers and toes. I also had serious night sweats that caused me to change my clothes numerous times each night. My body was just warm all the time, and I was constantly sweating. I was popping Zofran (an antiemetic) as if it were my job and trying to drink ginger ale, but nothing helped. I just kept looking at the clock and thinking, "If this is how I have to spend the next few months, I don't know how I'm going to get through this." My poor dog was so confused. He sat next to me cuddled up all night crying and wondering what was going on. Dogs really are the most loyal animals ever. Love ya, Justin!

Chemo Is Basically a Hangover

After venting to Dr. X all night, around four in the morning, I came to a serious conclusion: chemo is a lot like a hangover. Picture the worst hangover of your life, times five hundred. I went to one of the biggest party schools in New England, *and* I live in Miami, so I have serious experience with hangovers, which you would think would essentially make me a chemo pro. At UNH, we would play power hour with Mad Dog 20/20, play Edward Scissorhands and attach forty-ounce beers to both of our hands with tape, do keg stands with Franzia boxes of wine, and on and on. (Sorry to all my family members reading this.) We just did inappropriate things that you should not do and are so bad for your body—*so* many times. I'm completely fine with the possibility of not being able to have kids, because I was a very, very scary kid. I was such a jerk in college that I'm truly lucky to even be alive. Even in Miami during my younger years, I partied at nightclubs until five in the morning and then went home only to wake up a few hours later to continue the party on a boat (or throwing up off the side of it). In all actuality, I thought to myself, "My life is going to be a hangover, hopefully only until August, but I can do this! I survived all those times, and this is pretty much the same thing, right? Right." All jokes aside, going off on that "everything happens for a reason" tangent, I am almost convinced that my behavior in my early twenties prepared me for the beating that my body took during chemo and radiation.

If you don't or have never consumed alcohol, I can tell you that chemo is like the flu or a stomach bug times five hundred—minus the coughing and sneezing. You just feel fatigued, your heart races, you sweat, you're nauseous, and so forth. If you've ever gotten food poisoning to the point where you are dry heaving next to your toilet and can barely stand up, that's what chemo feels like, at first.

For cycle days two and three, I'm going to bunch them together. I had an etoposide infusion and prednisone both days. I took procarbazine chemo pills every night during that cycle. I basically had poison injected into me. Shout out to my chemo nurse: I can't remember your name, but thanks so much for telling me to start taking Compazine *before* chemo, and any time I felt nausea coming on. This absolutely *saved* my life, and I swear that this is the cure-all for chemo nausea. This and a boatload of water, and I'm OK. This really wasn't *that* bad. Other than that, I had (and still have) chemo brain like no other, and my taste buds were completely off. Even water tasted weird. Not a problem, though; at least I didn't get fat while I sat on my butt for six months.

Pain was a different story, though. The initial pain I experienced was from Neupogen shots I had to inject in my stomach. It felt like a shooting pain that rotated in random parts of my body, but it came and went. About seven to ten days after chemo, I became neutropenic (extremely low white blood cell count—neutrophils, in particular), which was tough because I couldn't be around people since I couldn't risk getting sick. I love my friends, but the worst part was not being able to touch my dog! I was in quarantine for about a week after the first chemo. If you wanted to come to my apartment, I would have to spray you with Lysol before you entered.

The last chemo of cycle two was on a Tuesday. That was one day of Bleomycin and Vincristine. These were push infusions. The premeds for this are what take so long. It feels like you're there forever. I think this one gave the weirdest feeling. You just feel loopy, like you're on another planet. Other than that, as long as I could manage the side effects, I was fine, and no one could even tell I was sick.

Talk Neutropenia to Me

Neutropenia is an abnormally low neutrophil (a type of white blood cell) count. Neutrophils comprise the majority of white blood cells and serve as the primary defense against infections by destroying bacteria in the blood. Neutropenia happens as a response to chemotherapy and typically occurs seven to ten days after treatment. When you are neutropenic, you are very susceptible to infection and must abide by the precautions set out by your oncologist/hematologist. I repeat: *must*! Your doctor prescribes injections such as Neupogen, which you inject into your abdomen for a prescribed number of days. The injections stabilize the neutrophil count. During the time you are neutropenic, you have to follow a specific diet. If my mom didn't ask to talk to a dietician before I was discharged from the hospital, I would have had no idea about this. So here are some tips for neutropenia:

Make sure not to eat out at restaurants during the time you are neutropenic, because you never know who's cooking with what and what bad bacteria might be in the food.

No sushi or anything raw.

No fresh fruit unless it has a peel on it. I ate only thick-skinned, fresh fruit such as bananas and oranges.

No fresh vegetables at all or anything with bacteria. You must wash your vegetables with vinegar and water before cooking them. Basically, everything has to be cooked.

No fresh flowers or plants, as they have too much bacteria.

Stay away from sick people! You don't want to catch what they have.

Always wash your hands and carry hand sanitizer.

Take your temperature frequently. If you have a temperature of 100.4 F or higher, go to the emergency room. Immediately! It doesn't matter if it's one o'clock in the morning—go!

Wear a mask if need be; you can't risk getting sick.

Avoid crowded areas.

Remember, chemo doesn't kill people. Infections do. Follow the diet and follow the protocol. Don't mess around when it comes to this.

Talk Side Effects to Me

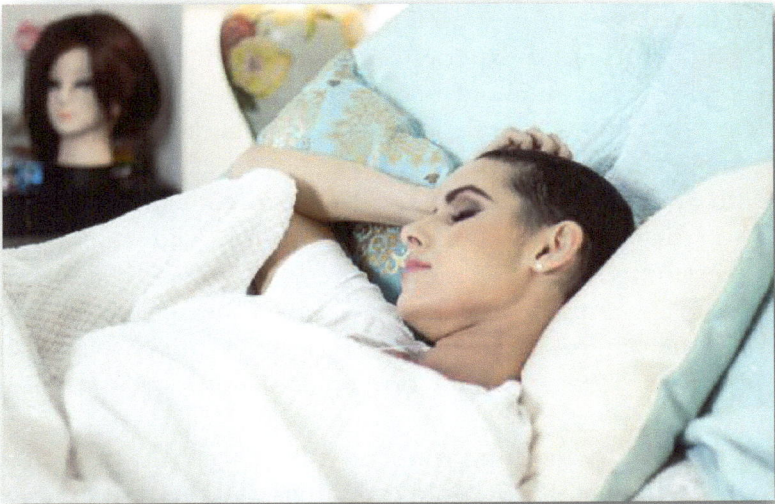

Nausea: I would become very nauseous before, throughout the entire treatment, and after chemo. I still randomly become nauseous. Zofran only worked for me during chemo through IV. During chemo, make sure you drink as much water as you can, and always bring a Gatorade to CTU as well. Ginger ale and crackers helped a bit. I would also get Ativan for my pre-med through IV during chemo, which helped a great deal with the nausea as well as the anxiety. But what really saved my life after CTU was Compazine. One of my chemo nurses recommended this to me, and it was the only thing that helped me. I would take it whenever I felt nausea coming on, basically every six hours. For most, it's trial and error with nausea medications, but don't feel like you have to live with the nausea. You don't. It's 2016, and there are many types of medications out there. Whoever tells you that the nausea can't go away is lying. Zofran didn't do a thing for me; however, Compazine worked for me. Metoclopramide is another drug that works for many. Controlling your nausea will make your journey so much easier. Make finding your nausea medication of choice your number-one priority. If you were just diagnosed and haven't started chemo yet, make sure you get the medications beforehand. I can also not stress enough to you how important it is to drink as much water as you can and stay hydrated. This will help with your side effects. I promise you.

Bone Pain: When I first started using Neupogen shots to increase my white blood cell count, I experienced intense bone pain. Take Claritin an hour before you are about to inject yourself with Neupogen. Mine went away eventually, but at first, it was bad and lasted a few hours. The Claritin helped a lot.

Mouth Sores and Pain: Ask your doctor for "Magic Mouthwash." It helps a ton. Swish it around in your mouth. It has lidocaine in it, so it numbs everything. Good-bye, mouth sores!

Bruising: I eventually looked like I'd been beaten with a bat, with bruises all over. There's really no way around this, but you can purchase an arnica roller to tone down the bruises. Probably the least of your worries, though.

Hair Loss: Sorry, nothing you can really do about this, unless you want to invest in one of those cold cap things, but they are super expensive. Check out my section on hair loss for more information.

Anxiety/Insomnia: My dosage of prednisone was extremely high. I couldn't sleep at all at first, and it also gave me major anxiety. Consult with your doctor and ask if you are able to take Benadryl or any over-the-counter sleep aid. This helped a lot for me and would make me fall asleep. Benzos (for anxiety) are extremely addictive, so you have to be careful with them, but in the case of cancer, you might need them. Klonopin was very helpful for me, especially at night, when I would get very anxious. I know many people are hesitant to go on antianxiety medications, but almost every person I know with cancer went on at least Zoloft, and it helped with anxiety and panic attacks. You can stop taking it when you're done with this life-changing journey. But it helps. Ativan is an absolute lifesaver and helps control the chemo-induced nausea as well. Remember, cancer is traumatic, so do what you need to do to get through it. It's temporary.

Neuropathy: My neuropathy started in my fingertips and then progressed throughout my hands. I found it to be the worst at night. I also had neuropathy in my feet. I didn't take anything for this, but I have heard from many of my cancer friends that Lyrica and Neurontin help a lot. Most of the time, it does go away after chemo. There is a chance, however, that it won't. It's a small price to pay for staying alive. Unfortunately, along with my neuropathy, I also developed foot drop (difficulty lifting the front part of the foot, which caused me to fall a lot). I did physical therapy for this and a muscle activation technique (MAT training). It eventually went away.

Chemo Brain: Chemo brain is a very common side effect from chemo and includes problems with memory and thinking. It's like a brain fog and causes cognitive dysfunction. This is completely normal, but I can't tell you any tricks or tips to deal with this because I almost just forgot what I was writing. Ha!

How I Personally Dealt with Chemo Pain

How did I deal with the pain from chemo? That is a common question with an easy answer. Unfortunately, my doctor didn't prescribe pain medication, because he's against it. I'm going to thank him for this because he helped give light to my journey. The pain I experienced on my off weeks of chemo made me feel more alive and invincible, and I used those feelings to empower me rather than to bring me down. I could have sat there and cried, which I never did. You would never see me cry during the off weeks. Ask my mom—never.

Instead, I would take my temperature at three in the morning to make sure I didn't have a fever and then carry on with how I deal with it—by telling my story to help other people. I created a blog, which I really think saved my life and helped many others. I documented everything I was going through. I believe my story can help save someone's life, but silence about my story only contributes to others' struggles. I don't post pictures, quotes, and selfies on my journey for attention. I got a lot of attention before my cancer—and trust me, I don't like attention; I used to run from it. I'm private. I'm confident with myself and know who I am. I don't need likes or followers to help tell me that. I genuinely want to help others who are going through the same thing know they will get through this. I want to raise awareness about cancer in general, because it's so easy for your life to take a 180; and while dealing with cancer is truly difficult, there are things that help.

Cancer fighters and survivors are the strongest people out there simply because they know they can survive whatever life throws at them. In a way, it's scary to me. I used to care about trivial things, and now, I think, if I ever go through a breakup, a friendship loss, a job loss, even a divorce in the future, it won't faze me as much. I know how to survive now, which can intimidate the rest of the world. I'll be able to carry on simply because I know I can. That's what lymphoma has taught me. You still have emotions, but at the same time, trivial things no longer affect you, and in many ways, you just don't give a f*ck. I can't see myself putting up with unacceptable behavior from anyone or anything going forward. Obviously, while going through cancer, you have many realizations. Now I carry on with my days without a second thought about things that would have upset me before. Lymphoma, you've kind of created a monster! But I mean, if your doctor does prescribe you pain pills because the pain is unbearable, you better pop those! Kidding. But seriously, do what works for you.

Talk Nurses to Me

I can't stress how important it is for you to become friendly with your nurses and to use them as a resource. They have seen it all and can often help you manage your symptoms, give you their thoughts and suggestions, or even just be there to listen. I became friends with several of the nurses who helped me out more than I could ever imagine. They see cases like yours daily, so they completely get it at a level on which your friends and family may not. Also, be prepared to wait at CTU for a long time. Sometimes chairs aren't available, and you'll have to wait for hours before one opens up for your treatment. So stock up on books, magazines, and movies; bring your iPad, and have things to do. Bring a blanket; it gets cold in there!

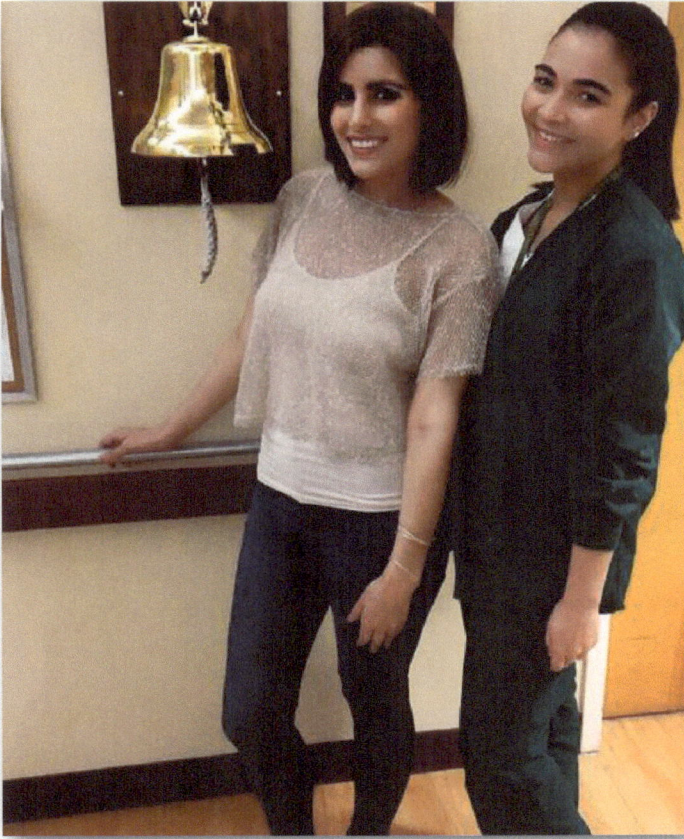

CHAPTER 3

Talk Cancer Treatment to Me: Now What?

There are probably a million things running through your mind right now.

Denial. You're still in denial. You look fine and don't understand how you can have cancer. You feel fine, and you feel like, "OK, I can do this." This is completely normal. Just know that your life is about to drastically change, and I mean drastically. The denial phase will wear off in a few weeks. For me, it wore off when my hair started falling out. At the beginning of your diagnosis, you're probably surrounded by friends and family, but when you go home, it becomes very real. Make sure to keep your friends and family very close. They are your support system and will help you get through this.

Freak-Out Mode. Depression and anxiety are likely. Very freaking likely. In fact, I'm going to be brutally honest with you and tell you that you will most likely experience both. Everyone reacts to cancer and chemo differently. This is how I reacted. There are two different categories of the freak-out mode: lifestyle change and hair loss. I'll go over both of them with you. This also includes extreme anger, which I will go over as well.

Keep in mind that this is coming from a single girl's perspective. One of my biggest concerns at the beginning was, "Oh my God; I have cancer. I'm damaged goods, and no one will ever want to date me! And I won't be able to have kids!" If you're thinking about the fertility aspect, don't worry. You have options. Worry about your health first, because if you are dead, you can't reproduce anyway.

As for being "damaged goods," I'm going to tell you what everyone else told me, and it's exactly true. You are not damaged goods! If anything, this journey will make you a badass warrior chick in high demand. Your stock is about to spike, sweetheart; trust me on this one. I've had men knocking at my door throughout this insane cancer journey, and I assure you this will happen to you too, as long as you follow my advice, of course! Men don't care that you have cancer. Let me rephrase that, *good men* don't care if you have cancer. The losers might care, and if they do, screw them! Would you really want to date someone who is shallow enough to care whether you have hair? Probably not. Other lifestyle changes include not being able to work, not being able to work out as much—or even at all, and social setting changes; but you will survive all of these. I cover these in later chapters.

Hair-Loss Freak-Out Mode. Most chemotherapy has the side effect of hair loss. For me, it came out strand by strand, two weeks after my first chemo. Then, every time I ran my hands through my hair, it would come out in chunks. I've had hair extensions basically my entire life, so for me, this was extremely hard. It's going to shed all over your apartment too. All over. All over your blankets, pillows, everywhere. It's mortifying. You have two options. You can go ahead and just shave your head so that you don't have to deal with your hair coming out in chunks—because believe me, it is traumatic as hell—or you can let it go until the last minute, and cut it day by day, which is what I did, initially. I had to stop chemo after my fourth cycle, to begin immediate radiation, because my cancer became refractory. All of my hair grew back within those two months. When I continued chemo, my hair fell out again, so I sucked it up and shaved it all off. It's up to you.

Talk Hair Loss to Me

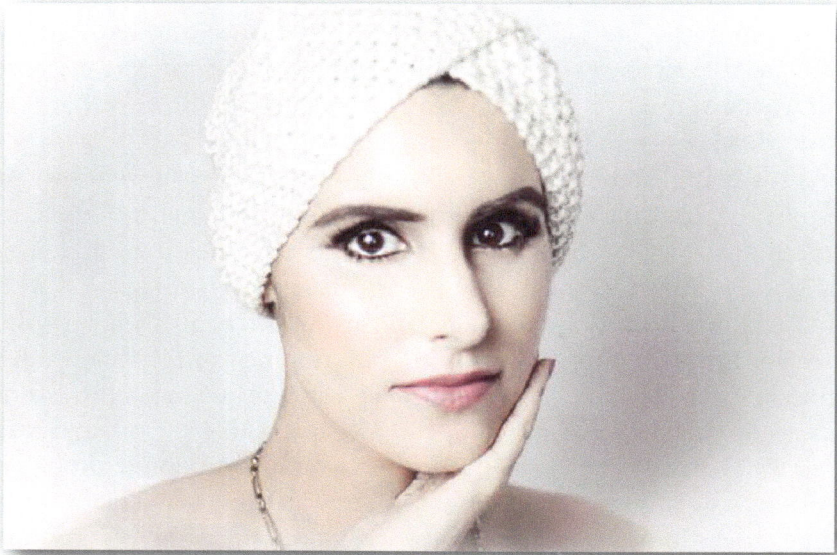

Losing your hair sucks. I'm not going to sugarcoat it; it's awful. As if feeling like crap from chemo isn't bad enough, having your hair fall out in chunks all over your floor and in your hands is not a fun feeling. About two weeks after I started chemo is when my hair first started to fall out. It went strand by strand, and then clump by clump, which might happen to yours too. I give major credit to all the women out there who immediately shaved their heads after diagnosis. I couldn't bring myself to do it, and I'm glad I didn't. Even though it was awful, and I waited until the last minute when I had no hair left. It helped me "experience" and take in my diagnosis more. It made it more real, and it made me feel more human.

Sometimes we need pain to feel alive. Even though it was hard, and I received daily clump-by-clump reminders of hair loss, I was fighting a huge battle, and in a sense, it made me feel brave. It made me feel like I was overcoming a major life change and that I would be stronger than anyone I knew after this. I thought of all my friends living normal lives, complaining about trivial things, and I'm over here fighting for my life. If I could survive this, I could survive anything. Even though it's just hair, it made me feel as if, when all this was over, I could truly take on the world. My goal was to be like Samantha from *Sex and the City*, and to rock the crap out of cancer, which is exactly what I did.

I remember hair loss was my main concern before I was discharged from the hospital. "Is my hair going to fall out, and when?" (Not logical concerns, such as what if I get an infection and end up in the hospital? What if I get lung disease or heart disease from the Bleomycin? What about my fertility? I'm pushing thirty over here, Doc.) I even tried convincing the on-call oncologist who discharged me that I wasn't going to lose my hair. Denial. He thought I was nuts. It's funny because during my first chemo cycle, I had one of my friends chop off my hair into a cute little bob. A week later, I went to my hematologist appointment. My hair looked *so* good, and I felt like I looked amazing for a cancer patient. I even ran into one of my respiratory techs from the ICU, and he was shocked at how good I looked. But my doc just looked at me, asking if I'd lost any hair yet. I said no. He knew it was coming, because when I got home it started falling out, strand by strand, and then in chunks.

It was hard, very freaking hard. In my opinion, I would take the nausea, the pain, the night sweats, the restless nights, and the anxiety together over losing my hair. This is just my opinion, and you are entitled to your own. My friend, Melissa, a fellow lymphoma survivor, kept telling me I would have fun with short wigs and head scarves. At the time I thought to myself, "This girl is out of her damn mind. There's no way I'm going to have fun wearing a wig and being bald." News flash! After six months and six cycles of chemo, I realized wigging out rocks! Depending on your insurance, you can submit this as a medical expense. Get a prescription from your provider, and your insurance may pay for it. So get at least one good wig and contact your insurance. Each wig costs a few hundred dollars. You can also buy a bunch of fun, cheaper, synthetic wigs online too. There are bunches of great websites that have affordable wigs for just fifty dollars (www.voguewigs.com is a good one—even eBay—there are so many options out there). My favorite wigs are any by Jon Renau. They are amazing and all look 100 percent real. I purchase them from www.galleryofwigs.com, I personally like the Zara, Kristen, and Drew models. Feel free to follow my blog, www.lymphomabarbie.

com, and if you like any of my wigs, of which I have more than I should, I will tell you where I got them.

The key with finding a good wig is to look for "full lace" or "lace front" so that it looks natural. I'm going to save you a lot of money right now. Go to your nearest wig store, try on a bunch of wigs, get the name and brand, and then you can most likely find them online for cheaper. Trust me, I'm talking about saving a minimum of $200. All my wigs are synthetic, so don't let someone try to sell you a human-hair wig for $4,500; they look and feel exactly the same. You can't tell that I have no hair with any of mine. I initially struggled with even putting my first wig on because I was so worried about what other people would think, and it scared me. Now I don't give a crap because no one can even tell! No joke, three cycles in, a nurse asked me how my hair had not fallen out yet. That's how real my wigs look. I rock the crap out of all my wigs, and it's so fun being able to change your look every day. Just go with it!

If you're a brunette, think about all the times that you've wanted to go blond but were scared to do so. And vice versa. Now you have your chance! You can have fun with head scarves too. There are so many cute styles to wear! Plus, you don't have to spend hours fixing your hair every day. Sorry to all my girlfriends out there, but my wigs look better than their real hair! All my friends joke about how my wigs look amazing all the time. Hands down, though, Jon Renau makes the best wigs ever—by far. They look better than my natural hair. Colorwise, the trick is to YouTube or Google the exact Jon Renau (or any other brand that you choose) color that you're looking for. A lot of people do wig reviews on YouTube, so there are videos showing the exact color and even style of the wig. Also, the wigs don't last that long, depending on how long you wear them. It's easy to refurbish them, though, with a steamer or a hot iron (Google "YouTube wig refurbishing"). I would suggest buying a longer one at first, and then just keep cutting it when it gets ratty to get the most bang for your buck.

Kylie Jenner rocks wigs daily and looks fabulous. It might take some time, but once you find a good wig or two, you will be golden, and you will have fun with it. Trust me on this one! This will help you get through chemo. I cannot express just how much this helped me get through chemo. When you look good, you feel good, and once you find your weaves, you will look amazing and be on the verge of kicking cancer in the booty! Oh, and don't forget to shave your head when there is nothing left, and you are ready to wear your wigs. You have to do this! Just a small warning: you might become addicted to buying wigs. The number I have in my closet is a bit scary.

As for your eyebrows and lashes, you might lose those too, which I did. I'm a big fan of the Anastasia Beverly Hills brand. You can buy a stencil to match the shape that you would like your brows to be. Fill them in with Brow Powder Duo, and then pencil in the rest with Brow Wiz. You can find this brand at Sephora, Nordstrom, Ulta, or online. If you lose your lashes, I'm a big fan of falsies, especially by MAC. I like the #33 because they look natural, or Ardell. If you're too lazy for this, try lining your lid with a brown eyeshadow, and then you can't even tell that you have no lashes. Boom!

So, in summary, the best products to purchase are these:

- Lace-front or full-lace wigs. Jon Renau has the most natural-looking wigs; the best styles are Zara, Kristen, and Drew. If you want to go shorter, I would suggest Kristen. It will last you the longest.
- Pricewise, Galleryofwigs.com is great for Jon Renau wigs.
- Anastasia Beverly Hills Brow Duo and Brow Wiz.

Extreme Anger

I can't tell you how angry I was during my treatment. I was angry at everyone around me: angry at all the doctors who failed to diagnose me on time, angry at my own doctor, angry at myself, and angry at people who I expected to be there for support but who couldn't have cared less. I didn't understand why this was happening to me and what I did to cause this. It's completely normal to be so angry at first because it's a lot to digest. It's healthy to be angry, but only for a certain amount of time. The key is to turn your anger into motivation to beat your cancer. Allow yourself to be angry at first, but then find something to help you deal with it. Writing and sharing my journey was a major anger relief for me. Other friends I have with cancer chose other things, like art, painting, photography, or do-it-yourself projects, and some even created cool jewelry lines. Do all the things you never had time for before (which are, of course, within the guidelines of what you're allowed to do when you are undergoing treatment). Now is your time!

Talk Friendships to Me

One of the hardest things you go through when you have cancer is realizing who cares about you, who doesn't, who never did, who is a good, genuine person, and who is not. At the beginning, people who you think would be part of your journey are nowhere to be found, and this is a hard truth you need to accept. At first you might become angered by this, but with time your "cancer brain," I like to call it, comes into play, and you just don't care. At all. It doesn't even faze you. I'm sure *every* single cancer patient and survivor can relate to this. It has nothing to do with you. Some people just suck. Once you realize that behavior like this is more about those people and not about you, you become free.

Unfortunately, you have to be wary because having cancer also attracts a lot of fake and opportunistic people around you. I can't tell you how many insincere people have reached out to me. People come out of the woodwork. They want to hang out and take pictures with the girl who has cancer and comment on social media posts to make themselves feel better or to look like a nice person on social media. Girls I haven't talked to in years who don't even like me—actually, they can't stand me—all tried to comment and reach out. People who just weren't even part of my crazy journey, or people who came to see me in the hospital and then disappeared, will suddenly want to hang out with you, especially if you make your journey public, like I did. Where were these people when I was in the hospital or stuck at home bedridden for six months struggling with chemo and radiation and relapses? You know who you are, and I definitely know who you are too.

People with cancer are smarter than you are. We've been through all the bullshit, and we see past it. We also won't think twice about you. Just know that we get what you're trying to do. It doesn't faze us. Don't even trip over these people. Your real friends will be revealed immediately. And you will be so thankful for cancer showing you who they actually are.

Change of Lifestyle Freak-Out

Many things you go through while dealing with cancer may seem, at the time, far worse than the cancer or chemo itself. Like everything else in life, the way that you handle these situations is all within your control and can make or break your situation. Life goes on with or without you, which is one of the toughest parts to accept when dealing with chemo. Your job goes on; your friends' lives go on; everything goes on; and this is usually the hardest thing to understand when you're going through treatment. Sometimes you miss out on important events, and it hurts.

For me, I had planned on being there for the birth of one of my best friend's babies. I was so excited for it, but I wasn't able to make it because I was neutropenic from chemo and couldn't be around anyone or risk getting an infection. (Again, chemo doesn't kill patients; infection is what kills.) I also wasn't able to go to Vegas for my sales meeting because I was in the hospital fighting for my life. And to top it all off, it was tough to have to be home all the time while my friends were all out living their lives. I felt like I was missing out on so much. While everyone else was having a good time, I was sitting in CTU getting injected with multiple different chemo drugs, and I'm only twenty-nine. Not exactly what I had signed up for.

I'm a very social person, and I love being out. For me it was hard to be home all the time. If I wasn't at home, I was at the cancer center getting scans or chemo, or I was at doctor appointments. Since I couldn't work, I knew I had to try to make my life seem as normal as possible, and I owe a *lot* of this to my friends. They came over all the time. We would have dinner dates, lunch dates, and so forth. I think this saved me and made me feel more like a normal person. I encourage anyone who is battling cancer—as hard as it is—try to go on with your normal life. It's easier said than done, but for me it helped more than anything. You might get really tired, but force yourself to do it! I remember going out with my friends to dinner until eleven. I was so exhausted from that and chemo that I slept until one in the afternoon the next day. And it's OK! It's easy to sit home, be sad, and feel bad for yourself, asking, "Why is this happening to me?" But as the weeks go by, you'll realize that cancer is both a curse and a blessing at the same time. At least for me it was. Mourning about your situation does nothing to change it, because trust me, I did my share of mourning. From my experience, getting out into the real world helped me feel a lot better than sitting at home crying.

Try to Live as Normally as Possible

I tried to live as normal a life as possible during treatment. So normal that sometimes I completely forget how sick I actually was. It's 50 percent mental. I met an amazing girl on Instagram who follows my blog, and she ended up living in Boston. My friend from Boston was visiting me, so I thought it would be perfect to have my friend deliver a small chemo care package to her before her first chemo session. I will never forget that as I was trying to write her a note, the neuropathy in my hands was so bad that I could barely write. To be honest, I couldn't write at all. For the first time in a while, it brought me to tears. I looked completely normal. You would never guess that I have cancer, but I was going through this battle that most who don't know me wouldn't even realize if they saw me on the street—or even understand, for that matter.

I let myself be sad for a few minutes and then moved on. That's what you have to do when you have cancer. You can let yourself be sad, and then you put one foot in front of the other, handle it, and move on. There is really no other way in my opinion. Chemo sucks. I'm not going to downplay it. As I wrote this, I was sitting in a chair, nauseous, attached to a machine that was administering a bag full of chemo through a port in my chest. This was happening while all my friends were at work. It was the beginning of my new sales quarter at work, and there was no place I would rather have been than in the field doing my job as a rep. It sucks, but sometimes you have to turn lemons into lemonade.

There is no point in sitting around bitching about how horrible your symptoms are, especially with other people. I'm going to tell you it's the worst thing you can do—to talk with other cancer patients who are very negative and only complain and contribute to negative energy. It will only make your symptoms worse. It helped to tell myself that things could always be worse. What if there weren't treatments available for cancer? As patients, we usually have options. Keep yourself occupied, handle it, fight, and move on. It will be over before you know it, I promise.

Change Your Way of Thinking

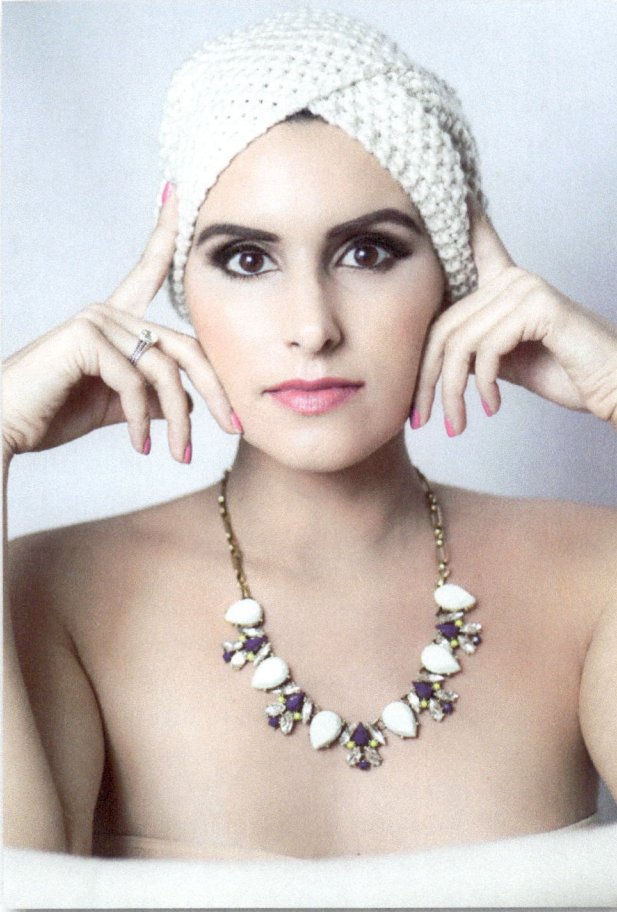

Just because you go through hell doesn't mean that you have to stay there. Whether you have cancer, you're sick, you've lost a friend, a family member, a job, even a significant other—you are responsible for how you handle your situation. You can let your situation destroy you or empower you. It's your choice. It's so easy to call it quits and just not get out of bed in the morning. Instead of dwelling on my situation, I saw it as God and the universe giving me time to myself to get rid of whatever it was that wasn't working for me.

I'm far from perfect, and I've made a lot of mistakes in life. I've taken a lot of things for granted, held unnecessary grudges and anger against people, and have acted like a spoiled brat. I've been inconsiderate of other people at times and very judgmental. I'm originally from Boston, and our values are completely different there than they are in South Florida. Over the past several years living in Miami, I've lost myself at times. I've been more focused on my looks and on other people's looks, rather than who a person is deep down inside—who I am deep down inside. I've been more concerned with whose yacht I'm going on and whose table I would be partying at than spending time developing meaningful relationships with significant people. I became so obsessed with working and making as much money as I could to buy materialistic items such as Rolex watches and Prada bags to impress people I didn't even know.

One of my best friends from work is a pharmaceutical rep also in Oklahoma. We are complete opposites; she's a Zen yogi and like a big sister who slaps sense into me every other day. She's always told me that, deep down inside, I'm not even close to whom I act like and that this city was making me lose myself. And she was totally right. Sometimes a city can consume you. I was acting like someone I wasn't, while on the side I was feeding homeless people and giving food to stray animals on the street. My manager once found dog food in my glove compartment during a field ride, and I admitted to him that *sometimes* when I see stray animals during work hours, I detour to Petco and buy food to feed them. Sorry, A! And one of my doctor's offices has yelled at me multiple times for feeding stray cats outside their office (sorry, but I'll continue to do that when I get back to work. Ha!). I even completed training to be a wish granter for the Make-A-Wish Foundation before my diagnosis. That is who I really am. I don't know why I was afraid to show it. So now I had room to rebuild. I had room to figure out what I want in life and who I want to be. And this cancer journey helped me do exactly that.

Above all, I want to be known and remembered as the girl who took a shitty situation and turned it into gold. I want to help not only cancer fighters but also people in general to be able to change their outlooks on life. I want to be able to help you, reading this. But I can only help you so much. Your attitude will be everything during this process, and your thoughts become truth. The more you dwell, the worse your situation will become.

Treat This as a Blessing in Disguise

I used to hate celebrating my birthday before lymphoma. I was dreading turning twenty-nine because it was one year closer to thirty, one year closer to society expecting you to be living your life a certain way. As my friend Melissa, a fellow lymphoma survivor, said to me, "After you fight for your life, every year that you're alive means so much more." So this year was my best birthday yet.

I don't wish cancer upon anyone. It's a horrible monster, and I hope that one day we don't have to call ourselves survivors or talk about remission. I hope that one day we can find a cure. I hope that one day people like myself, and others who have it worse than I do, don't have to worry about relapsing, getting chemotherapy-induced secondary malignancies, and going through all this again. I truly believe that with all of the talented oncologists and hematologists out there, we will one day find a cure.

In March, after being diagnosed, I remember telling myself there was a reason why this was all happening to me. Doctors say they can't tell their patients why they get cancer because no one knows and there is no reason why it happens to any specific person. So in a twisted way, I thank God for allowing me to fight this battle and for waking me up. Lymphoma shook me up like hell. It made me face reality and take my life into my own hands. It gave new meaning to my life, and in some messed-up way, it was the best thing that ever happened to me. Without going through this battle, I wouldn't be the person who I am right now typing this. I've learned more about myself in the last six months than I've learned in the last twenty-nine years of life. You will learn a ton about yourself and about how strong you really are. You will ultimately become stronger than anyone you know. Trust that.

Realize What's Really Important

Lymphoma made me realize what is truly important, and whatever cancer you might have will help you realize that too. It's helped me grow in all the places I never thought I would. I've always known I have amazing friends, but I can't even begin to express how lucky I am even to have the privilege of knowing all my friends. All of my best friends from Boston, from work, and college really stepped up beyond belief. You all know who you are, and you hold such a special place in my heart.

My Miami friends, I'm also so lucky to have you all. Especially seeing as how Miami is such a transient city, and it's so hard to find genuine friends, I'm lucky to say I have a solid group of about twenty of you, and you're the best people I've ever met in my life. I don't need to name drop everyone because you all know who you are. You all made me feel so normal, never made me feel like I was sick, and still made me feel beautiful and like my old self, even with no hair. And I thank lymphoma for rekindling friendships too. Life is busy, and sometimes we lose touch with people because we're so preoccupied with our own lives. It's amazing how you can just pick up right where you left off with certain people. I'm so glad I've become so close with so many new friends too. And with people who I met only recently who I can truly say are best friends of mine now. Never glorify the term "busy." There is *always* time, and if you don't make it now, you will regret it later. Trust me.

Learn to Let Shit Go

Cancer teaches you to truly let shit go. I'm thankful to lymphoma for teaching me to let trivial things go and for reintroducing people into my life with whom I've had stupid fallings-out. When something tragic happens to you, you realize who matters and who doesn't. When you're sitting in a hospital bed or attached to a bag of chemo fighting for your life, you're going to regret getting into stupid arguments and losing touch with people for stupid reasons. You're going to regret the he said–she said bullshit. News flash…*none* of that shit matters when you're on the verge of life or death!

God works in miraculous ways by bringing people back into your life at the perfect time. But the most important thing while dealing with cancer is to realize *who is genuine* and *who is not.* Not all friendships or re-lationships are meant to be rekindled just because you or someone else is sick. Sometimes you have to cut people out of your life because they are toxic to you and don't make you a better person. You have to take responsibility for how—on good or bad terms—you leave those relation-ships. It's something we all have to carry with us forever.

It is inappropriate and by *no* means OK to reach out to someone in an extremely insincere manner simply to help *you* feel better for being a mean person in the past—a straight-up bully out of an episode of *Mean Girls,* saying mean, hurtful things about another person. I found that this happened a lot to me. Old friends who had been so horrible and just downright inhumane to me in the past wanted to reach out. I even had an ex-boyfriend show up at the hospital and reach out to me in the most textbook-style insincere way. He would ask me how I was doing, and when I told him, he would completely disregard it. He reached out to make himself feel better for being a crappy person to his ex-girlfriend who was then on the verge of life or death. He then felt so dumb by his behavior, that he blocked every single mutual friend that we had in common, as well as myself, on social media. Unfortunately for some, people will forget what you said but never forget how you made them feel. People with cancer, we don't buy the BS. We realize who is real and who is fake. We are smarter than you. Life is short. Move on, and let that shit go! Fix yourself first.

Lymphoma has taught me more than I can ever imagine and has made me such a strong person in the process. I truly believe your cancer will do the same for you. It will introduce you to amazing doctors and nurses you would have never met otherwise. You will learn a lot, and you will learn fast. Lymphoma, you've taught me a ton. You've helped me realize that tomorrow isn't promised and that every day is a gift. You've taught me that everyone I meet is fighting a battle I know nothing about—just like I was—and to always be kind. You've taught me not to care about materialistic or superficial things, because at the end of the day, none of that crap matters, especially if you don't have your health. Without your health, you have nothing. You taught me to not take crap from anyone (not like I did before, but I'm on another level now, which is pretty frightening. Ha!) and not to care what *anyone* thinks of me—which I can truly say, I am now able to do! You taught me that even though I can't control what life throws at me, I *can* control how I handle it and how I react to it, and I think this is so important. It doesn't matter what happens to you; what matters is how you handle it. Whenever I start doubting myself, I think of how far I've come, all the fears I've overcome, and this crazy battle. The most important thing I've learned from all this is always to hang in there no matter how hard things get, because it can take a *very* short time for wonderful things to happen!

Find a Cancer Army

Chemo has a way of sneaking up on you. It's an understatement to say that one day you feel good and the next you feel horrible. I can't tell you how many times I awoke at two in the morning, drenched in sweat, to shooting pain so unbearable, it almost made me physically sick. Guess what? There are thousands of people just like you going through the same thing that you can connect with on social media. There is a hashtag on Instagram called #noonefightsalone, and it's absolutely true: no one fights alone. There are days when you feel mentally and physically weak. You look in the mirror and can't even recognize yourself because chemotherapy has destroyed who you once were on the outside. You cry and let yourself be down for a bit, ask God why this is happening to you, then you move on with your day. No one fights alone. Although there are days when I have felt more alone than I've ever felt in my life, there are millions of people going through the exact same physical and emotional journey as I was. I've connected with so many people through social media who are experiencing everything I experienced throughout this crazy cancer journey. You are not alone. Throughout the world, cancer connects people in a strange way.

Search Instagram for hashtags of your type of cancer, and reach out to people who are posting pictures and quotes. They are going through the same thing, or have been through it, and will be more than willing to help and empathize with you. There are also support groups on Facebook. To be honest, I wasn't a huge fan of these, because I found them to be extremely negative, and that's the last thing I wanted to pop up on my newsfeed. However, if you see someone posting positive messages, befriend that individual. That's who you need in your army. Message people on Instagram, connect with them on Facebook, and build your army! You will be very surprised at how many people are going through the exact same thing as you are. I've met so many people through Instagram whom I talk to daily. Megan, I heart you girl and I can't wait to meet you so soon! I can't stress how important it is to find your cancer army. Yes, you probably have a support system of friends and family, but unless they have or have had cancer, as much as they would like to, they can't relate to certain things that you are going through.

CHAPTER 4

Real Cancer Talk—No BS

Talk Timing to Me

'll never forget the weekend when I was taking a walk with my dog. After four cycles of chemo, the neuropathy in my hands became almost unbearable and had spread to my legs, making it extremely difficult even to walk. (I eventually found out I had foot drop, a side effect of Vincristine.) While trying to walk a half mile, I managed to fall to the ground three times. Four cycles of escalated chemo later, the side effects were officially a b*tch. Real talk—the side effects from chemo are no joke. So what did I do? I picked myself up off the ground and continued walking. When you know how it feels to be stuck in an ICU fighting for your life, you learn that even walking is a luxury and that it could always be so much worse, so I figured out a way to deal with these side effects. I started muscle-activation techniques (MAT) at my friend's gym.

The main questions I found myself asking throughout my journey were all along the lines of "What if?" What if I'd been diagnosed earlier? What if the allergist had realized I didn't have allergies? What if my PCP had put all my symptoms together and realized I had lymphoma two years ago? It's so easy to become angry and trip over the what-ifs, when in reality, in my opinion, everything happens for a reason, and you have to trust in God's timing. Although it stinks that I could have been in treatment for stage I or II lymphoma, rather than IV, I look back and think, "If I would have been diagnosed two years ago, I wouldn't have been prepared to handle a situation like this."

Two years ago, my mind-set had been completely different. I was negative, completely lost, and unhappy with my job. I was hanging out with the wrong crowd and was in a relationship that just wasn't a good fit for me. If I were to have faced cancer two years ago, I would have been emotionally screwed, which would have led my being physically screwed too, because like I said, cancer is 50 percent how you choose to handle it. If I'd had to rely on some of my friends at the time, or the person who I was in a relationship with to support me during such an ordeal, I would have been sh*t out of luck! I was hanging out with so many of the wrong people. My priorities were all mixed up. I hung out with people who would tear me down instead of build me up. People who only cared about partying and going to events to be seen. Women that only cared about how much money a man had, and traveling for free, rather than what else that man had to offer other than his money. People who were jealous and envious. I was caught up dating the wrong person for way too long. When my aunt passed away, my ex-boyfriend had been more concerned about networking at a barbecue and partying with his friends in NYC, rather than supporting someone who had been so close to him for so long. I can't even imagine how I would have been supported during what I've gone through in the past six months. To this day, this man is so selfish, opportunistic, negative, and just not a good person. He is someone who will smile to your face, then bad mouth you behind your back ; a user of other people, who only cares about reaching his way to the top, even at the expense of others. I thank God every day that this person was removed from my life, but I did learn a lot from him. I learned exactly the type of person that I would never want to be. But like me, he has his own path to take and his own lessons to learn in life, including learning that some behaviors are in no way conducive to having meaningful connections with others. This goes for friends that I had at the time too.

But we live and learn, and I truly believe there are no coincidences in life. People enter and exit our lives for a reason. At the time, it's hard to see the reason, but everything is a learning experience. Timing is everything. I think about it now, and although yes, my situation is annoying, I'm prepared for it. The people who have come into my life within the past few years, even the past year, have made my cancer journey so much easier. From my coworkers who have become best friends, to new friends, and of course, old friends, I wouldn't have the motivation I do now to beat this crazy monster!

It's very strange how God has specific people enter our lives when we really need them. In my situation, he had Dr. X enter it when things were really rough at the beginning and until I was mentally able to get it together and handle my situation. God also strengthened my friendships with every other person in my life too, leading to an amazing support system, which is key to beating cancer. So you can keep asking yourself why this is happening to you and why you were diagnosed at the time you were. Most of the time, the answers are right below the surface. Keep digging, and you will eventually find them!

Talk Setbacks to Me

Setbacks. Waiting. Setbacks are such an overlooked part of our cancer journeys, which can leave you an emotional wreck. Traumatic events in our lives, such as cancer, leave scars—physical and emotional scars—but sometimes it's in the silent hours that we are really able to see them. And I think our scars are what ultimately keep us going.

Often during chemo, your white blood cell count goes so low that you become neutropenic, and you have to stop chemo and take shots to boost your white blood cell count before you can continue with chemo again. No, not fireball shots (I wish). Neuopogen shots in your belly. It can take days, even weeks, to get your count back up. This is what makes your heart stop—when your doctor tells you that you have to hold off on chemo. Every cancer patient literally counts the day of each cycle and when it will be over with. My chemo was really strong, so my WBCs always got crazy low. My life during chemo revolved around being neutropenic, but my doctor said f*ck it and let the nurses continue to blast me with chemo because he wanted that cancer O-U-T, and so did I. See ya!

In radiation, thrombocytopenia (Look at those big words I'm learning! I should totally be an oncology drug rep. Then maybe I'll be able to marry an oncologist!) is a delay I faced for about three weeks during treatment. My platelet counts were much too low to continue radiation because the radiation had blasted the crap out of me. Continuing treatment with low platelets can cause internal, as well as external, bleeding.

I had pretty much reached the halfway point of radiation hell and had to stop because my platelets were too low. So I got my blood tested every other day, cried to my nurse, Vanessa, when they told me to go home because the platelet count was too low, called my mom and sobbed, and rinsed and repeated—mainly because I was so over it and just wanted it done. I think I'm the only psycho patient who actually demanded blood infusions.

The waiting part and the setbacks until you can resume treatment are by far one of the worst parts of the whole process. They force you to take everything in. When you're in treatment, you're either so sick, sleeping, so busy at the cancer center and so focused on getting this crap over with, that you don't really have time to think and let your scars set in. It's so easy to get upset during the setbacks. You think of all the hell you have been through, and, honestly, it makes you second-guess if you can make it through. Hell. Literally hell. Being cut open, burned, and poisoned equals hell. You think about how much you have been through, physically and emotionally, and no one truly gets it, unless that person has been there or has been a caregiver to someone with cancer. Your nurses, however, totally get it. Your doctors? I'm not so sure! They just want to treat you.

I hope all of my favorite residents are reading this, so you know what it feels like to be in the patient's shoes. You don't learn that in med school. You learn it from your annoying patient who bugs you every day! Ha! Your friends and family always mean well, but there is nothing—and I repeat, nothing—more annoying than people telling you, "Be strong." There comes a point when you've been so strong for so long that you just break. Let me be weak. It's OK to be weak. This is what I love about my mom. She never told me to be strong because she knows I'm strong. She reminded me where I have been, how far I've come, that I have a plan, and that it could always be so much worse. Always be so much worse.

I think our scars, the pain, and how messed up these types of situations get us are what really keep us going. All the setbacks, all the side effects, and all the bullshit that we deal with on a daily basis—our baggage. As many times as you want to give up, at the end of the day when you're sitting on your couch crying because you relapsed, or you can't get your treatment and have to hold off, it just shows you how much crap you have been through and makes you step up. And I think one of the most amazing parts of this journey is that, yes, you have a support system, but at the end of the day, *you* are the one who has to deal with everything.

So many women and men in my generation rely on the opposite sex to "complete" them. It almost makes me feel sorry for these people in a way, because in life, at the end of the day, you have to learn to be complete on your *own* and not be defined by another person. Cancer forces you to be complete on your own and to be able to pick up your *own* broken pieces. And carry on. Having someone on top of this is just a bonus. That's the point of the scars; they keep you going. They show you that once you've been through hell, life will be a breeze. It has to be. So don't trip over the setbacks. Allow yourself to cry, allow yourself to be down, and then put one foot in front of the other and try to keep going. Find a side project that you have always wanted to complete, that you never really had the time to do. During my three-week setback, I redecorated my entire house. Literally. The do-it-yourself projects kept me busy, and I finally had a cool spot to relax in while going through all this crap! I also watched every Netflix show and movie possible.

CHAPTER 5

Talk Radiation to Me

Burn, Baby, Burn

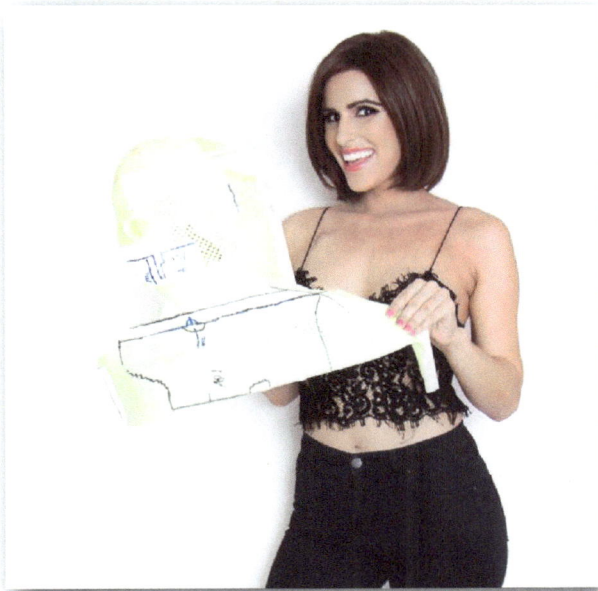

So you've finished chemo, and now you're on to radiation. Radiation treats cancer with high-energy waves to kill your tumors. In my case, we treated areas rather than the exact tumors. So my neck, chest, abdomen, and spleen were treated. Before treatment, you go through CT simulation, where your team makes you a mask that covers your head and neck, and they determine which areas they'll treat. When you begin radiation, you and your mask are strapped onto a table so you can't move. Radiation treatment involves essentially burning the crap out of your body in hopes of eliminating the cancer. Usually, radiation is last in your treatment regimen. In my case, the protocol was switched up. After my fourth cycle of chemo, a few new spots of cancer popped up, and my doctor was extremely worried about my spleen, so I started immediate radiation and then returned to finish my chemo.

My first radiation was a big WTF moment for me. I was strapped onto a table, with the mask hurting like heck, and I couldn't breathe out of my mouth, only through my nose. When you're in there, you don't feel a thing. You just hear noises and see a machine that looks like a spaceship rotating around you. The trippy thing is that you can't move, and you're stuck there for forty-five minutes to an hour. So you end up contemplating life and how, at twenty-nine years old, your entire body is literally being burned. That's fine. Heads up! If you're claustrophobic, take antianxiety medication beforehand, because it's really weird at first, and the mask is uncomfortable. But you will eventually get used to it! The first session is the worst.

The most important thing to tell yourself during this journey is that God *never* gives you more than you can handle. *Ever.* All those moments in life when you didn't think you would make it through, you made it through. You can ask, "Why me?" every day of your treatment. I do it occasionally too, but then I realize, why not me? It's hard as hell, but I can handle it. God doesn't give cancer or hardships to *weak* people—simply because they couldn't handle it. Cancer fighters and survivors are some of the strongest people out there because they know deep down that they can survive. Every single person I know who is currently fighting cancer or who has fought cancer just has a different swagger. (Sorry, I hate that word but can't think of a different one thanks to chemo brain!) Not even just cancer, but people who have faced hardships in general. I don't know one person who is a single mom or dad, who's been through a messy divorce, who's lost a friend or a family member, who has a disease or illness, or who had a rough childhood who *isn't* a strong person. These are the kind of people I look up to—the ones who simply man up and carry on. They are my motivation to man up and carry on because playing the victim card is way too easy, and I don't do easy. I have no desire to be whiny because of my situation, and I don't want anything handed to me. I think that this journey will ultimately make us stronger than we already are.

It's hard—very hard. I'm not trying to downplay this. But at the end of the day, my doctors have a plan. And yours will most likely have plans for you too. Whether those plans work or not is in God's hands, but they have a plan. And I have a plan for myself too, whenever this ordeal is over. My plan is never to take anything for granted—not one thing. To live in the moment, not worry about tomorrow, and to actually *live*. So if you're going through hell, keep going. It's almost over.

Radiation Tips and Tricks

Everyone handles chemo and radiation differently. For me, radiation was pretty bad—until I was able to learn how to manage it, that is. The two main side effects of radiation for me were nausea and vomiting. After dealing with these bad boys for two weeks, I figured out the tips and tricks to prevent these from happening; they're not fun!

- Drink enough water each day to prevent dehydration. Drink as much water as you can.
- Ask your doctor to prescribe you an antinausea medication. You should take it before radiation and whenever else your doctor recommends. It's 2016, so they *do* have medications to help with this. You just have to test to find out which one(s) work for you (for examp
- le, Compazine, Zofran, and so on). For me, Zofran did nothing. Compazine helped a lot.
- To ease the pain of swallowing, take two Extra Strength Tylenol forty-five to sixty minutes before you eat a meal. I know how impossible it is even to try to swallow food, and this saved my life. It's still tough, but it helps a ton! If this doesn't work for you, ask your doctor for something stronger. Chloraseptic spray also helps.

- Eat five to six small meals instead of three large ones. This will help settle your stomach. I like to make shakes. I make one in particular that I love: blend one banana, a little bit of oatmeal, some water or milk, and one scoop each of peanut butter and protein powder. It goes down very easily.
- Eat and drink very slowly, and don't lie down right after eating.
- Avoid eating greasy, fried, or spicy foods. Don't eat foods that are too hot or too cold.

Shout out to Dr. Markoe for this awesome list. Below are the foods I found to be very easy on my stomach and easy to swallow even when I had severe throat pain or difficulty swallowing:

- Chicken, vegetable, or beef broth
- Ginger ale
- Pedialyte, especially if you are vomiting
- Water
- Tea
- Ensure (it's also packed with vitamins and nutrients your body needs)
- Oatmeal
- Noodles
- Soft potatoes, no skin
- White rice
- White toast
- Popsicles
- Yogurt
- Canned fruit
- Pasta with white sauce only and cheese
- All cold cereal, but wait till it gets soggy, and then throw in some bananas
- Any soups, except tomato based

Avoid vinegar, lemon, or anything very acidic; cheese with jalapeño peppers; and carbonated beverages. If you're going to drink ginger ale, make sure it goes a bit flat.

Sometimes during radiation, your platelets become too low to continue, which I discussed earlier in the section on setbacks. While doctors say there is no way to boost your platelets, I did a little research and found things that I believe helped boost mine. Even though every doctor will probably disagree with this, these little tricks worked! My nurses agreed too. Ha!

- Papaya! Buy some papaya juice. Fresh is always better. Have a few glasses a day. For me, this helped, despite popular belief that it doesn't do anything.
- Eat a lot of spinach and kale. I would make smoothies with spinach, kale, banana, and orange juice. They are delicious too.
- Wheat grass. This is high in chlorophyll. I would have one wheatgrass shot a day, which you can purchase at a local juice bar or at Whole Foods, if there is one in your area.
- Pumpkin is another food that is rich in vitamin A, which is said to help support platelet development.

CHAPTER 6

And That's a Wrap!

Talk Kicking Cancer's Booty to Me

I hope I've gone over the majority of things you will need to know for your journey. It can also be very helpful to reach out directly to the association that applies to your specific cancer for more resources. For example, if you have leukemia or lymphoma, the Leukemia and Lymphoma Society offers a great deal of helpful information to patients, including books on your disease, support systems, and even a co-pay assistance program, if you are eligible.

If you've finished reading this, then congratulations; you're officially on the road to kicking cancer in the booty! These tips and tricks are what helped me survive my journey and are based on my own personal experience. Everyone experiences cancer, chemotherapy, radiation, and side effects differently. I hope sharing my struggle and giving you tips helps give you the strength you need to fight yours. Always remember that no one fights alone. There are tons of people going through the same thing all across the world. Take care for now, and keep fighting. You have a big team behind you, including me! Oh and PS- on August 18, 2016, after seven long months, I have finally entered remission and have no evidence of disease.

Author Biography

Jessica Lynne DeCristofaro was twenty-eight when she was diagnosed with Stage IV B Hodgkin's Lymphoma. After receiving her diagnosis and leaving the hospital, she found that no real guidebook for cancer sufferers existed. So she resolved to create one.

Starting a blog, *Lymphoma Barbie*, to chronicle her own cancer journey, she was so touched by people's responses that she expanded her writings into a book.

DeCristofaro, a graduate of the University of New Hampshire, lives in Miami, Florida, where she works as a pharmaceutical sales representative.

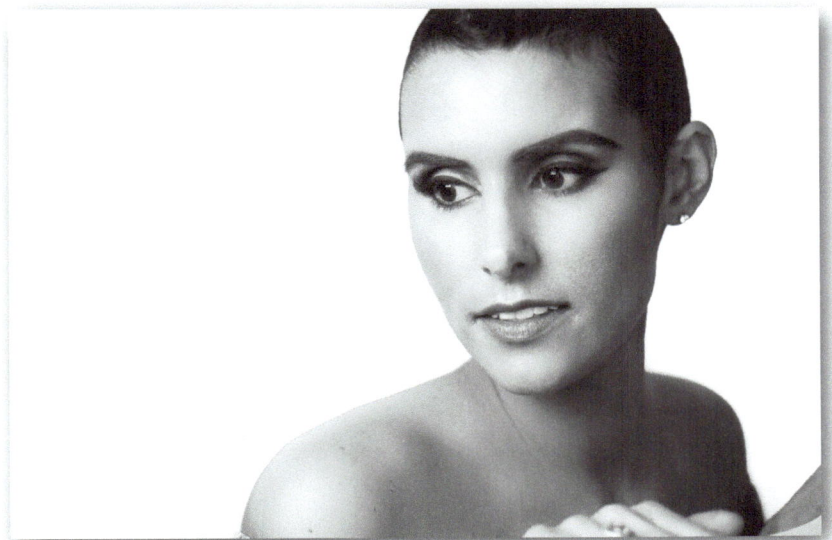